Healthy Habits for a Better Life

A comprehensive guide to achieving optimal health and wellness

By
Brown A. Rodriguez

Table of Content

Chapter 10: The role of technology and digital tools in tracking and promoting healthy habits

Chapter 1: **The importance of healthy habits in achieving optimal health and wellness**

Introduction:

Healthy habits are crucial in achieving optimal health and wellness. These habits not only help in preventing various diseases but also contribute to a happier and more fulfilling life. In this comprehensive guide, we explore the importance of healthy habits and how they can impact our overall well-being.

1. Exercise: Regular exercise is essential for maintaining physical health. It helps in keeping the heart and lungs functioning properly, building strength and flexibility, and reducing the risk of chronic diseases such as heart disease, diabetes, and obesity. Engaging in physical activity for 30 minutes or more, five days a week, can

greatly improve one's health and wellness.

2. Nutrition: A balanced and nutritious diet is another crucial component of healthy living. Eating a variety of foods that are high in vitamins, minerals, and nutrients can improve overall health, boost energy levels, and prevent chronic diseases. It is important to limit the intake of processed foods, saturated fats, and added sugars, and to instead focus on eating fresh fruits and vegetables, whole grains, lean protein, and healthy fats.

3. Sleep: Getting adequate sleep is crucial for both physical and mental health. Lack of sleep can result in a range of health issues, including a weakened immune system, fatigue, and an increased risk of chronic diseases. Aiming for 7-9 hours of

quality sleep each night can help improve overall health and well-being.

4. Stress Management: Chronic stress can take a toll on both physical and mental health. Engaging in stress-reducing activities such as meditation, yoga, or exercise can help reduce stress levels and improve overall wellness. Taking breaks and practicing self-care is also important for managing stress and promoting health.

5. Avoiding Harmful Habits: Avoiding harmful habits such as smoking, excessive alcohol consumption, and drug use is crucial for maintaining optimal health. These habits can lead to a range of health problems, including heart disease, cancer, and liver disease.

Conclusion:

In conclusion, healthy habits are a fundamental part of achieving optimal health and wellness. By incorporating exercise, nutritious eating, adequate sleep, stress management, and avoiding harmful habits into our daily routine, we can greatly improve our overall well-being and lead a happier and more fulfilling life. This comprehensive guide serves as a roadmap to help you adopt healthy habits and achieve optimal health and wellness.

Chapter 2: **How to make healthier food choices and develop a balanced diet**

Introduction:

Making healthier food choices and developing a balanced diet are essential components of a healthy lifestyle. In this comprehensive guide, we explore the steps you can take to make healthier food choices and develop a balanced diet that meets your nutritional needs.

1. Understanding Nutritional Requirements: The first step in making healthier food choices is to understand your nutritional requirements. This includes knowing your daily calorie needs and the recommended intake of macronutrients (carbohydrates, protein, and fat) and micronutrients (vitamins and minerals). By

understanding your nutritional needs, you can ensure that your diet is balanced and meets all of your nutritional requirements.

2. Planning Meals: Planning your meals in advance can help you make healthier food choices. Start by making a grocery list of nutritious foods, including fresh fruits and vegetables, lean proteins, and whole grains. Avoid processed foods and snacks high in sugar and fat. By having healthy options readily available, you can make healthier food choices when you're hungry.

3. Eating a Variety of Foods: Eating a variety of foods can help ensure that you get all the nutrients your body needs. Aim to include a variety of fruits and vegetables, whole grains, lean proteins, and healthy fats in your diet. Experiment with new foods and

recipes to keep your diet interesting and satisfying.

4. Portion Control: Portion control is an important aspect of a balanced diet. Eating larger portions can lead to weight gain, while smaller portions can help you maintain a healthy weight. Use smaller plates and bowls to help control portions, and aim to eat slowly, savoring each bite, to help you feel full faster.

5. Limiting Processed Foods and Added Sugars: Processed foods and snacks high in sugar and fat can be high in calories and low in nutrients. Limiting these foods in your diet can help you maintain a healthy weight and reduce your risk of chronic diseases such as heart disease, diabetes, and obesity.

6. Incorporating Healthy Fats: Healthy fats, such as those found in nuts,

seeds, avocados, and olive oil, are an important part of a balanced diet. They help to keep you feeling full and satisfied, and they provide energy for your body. Aim to include healthy fats in your diet, but limit saturated and trans fats, which can raise cholesterol levels and increase your risk of heart disease.

Conclusion:
In conclusion, making healthier food choices and developing a balanced diet is essential for achieving optimal health and wellness. By following the steps outlined in this comprehensive guide, you can ensure that your diet is balanced, nutritious, and meets all of your nutritional needs. By adopting these habits, you can take control of your health and lead a happier and more fulfilling life.

Chapter 3: **The benefits of regular exercise and tips for creating a fitness routine**

Introduction:

Regular exercise is one of the most important components of a healthy lifestyle. In this comprehensive guide, we explore the numerous benefits of regular exercise and provide tips for creating a fitness routine that works for you.

1. Physical Health Benefits: Regular exercise has numerous physical health benefits, including reducing the risk of chronic diseases such as heart disease, diabetes, and obesity. Exercise can also improve cardiovascular health, build strength and flexibility, and increase energy levels.

2. Mental Health Benefits: Regular exercise can also have a positive

impact on mental health. It can reduce stress and anxiety, improve mood, and enhance cognitive function. Exercise has been shown to have a positive effect on depression and can even help prevent cognitive decline in older adults.

3. Weight Management: Regular exercise can help with weight management by burning calories and building muscle. Incorporating both aerobic exercise (such as running or cycling) and strength training into your fitness routine can help you achieve and maintain a healthy weight.

4. Finding an Exercise You Enjoy: To make exercise a habit, it is important to find an activity that you enjoy. This could be anything from dancing to yoga to playing a sport. By finding an activity that you enjoy, you are more

likely to stick with it and make it a regular part of your routine.

5. Setting Realistic Goals: Setting realistic goals is an important step in creating a fitness routine. Start by setting achievable goals, such as exercising for 30 minutes a day, three days a week. As you progress, you can gradually increase the intensity and duration of your exercise.

6. Incorporating Variety: To avoid boredom and keep your fitness routine interesting, it is important to incorporate variety into your workouts. Try different activities, switch up your routines, and experiment with new exercises to keep your body challenged and engaged.

7. Making Time for Exercise: Finding time for exercise can be a challenge, especially for those with busy

schedules. Incorporating physical activity into your daily routine, such as walking or biking to work, can make it easier to fit exercise into your day. You can also consider working out at home or using online resources for convenient and flexible workout options.

Conclusion:
In conclusion, regular exercise is an essential component of a healthy lifestyle. By incorporating exercise into your daily routine, you can reap numerous physical and mental health benefits, achieve and maintain a healthy weight, and lead a happier and more fulfilling life. The tips provided in this comprehensive guide will help you create a fitness routine that works for you, allowing you to adopt healthy habits and achieve optimal health and wellness.

Chapter 4: **The role of sleep in overall health and tips for getting better sleep**

Sleep is a vital component of overall health and wellness, yet it is often overlooked in the pursuit of a healthier lifestyle. Many people believe that they can get by on limited sleep and compensate by eating well and exercising regularly. However, the truth is that getting sufficient, high-quality sleep is essential for physical and mental health. In this article, we will explore the role of sleep in overall health and provide tips for getting better sleep.

The Role of Sleep in Overall Health

Sleep plays a crucial role in many physiological processes that are critical for our health and well-being. During sleep, the body repairs and rejuvenates cells and tissues, regulates hormones, and consolidates memories. It also helps to maintain a healthy immune system and reduces the risk of chronic diseases such as obesity, diabetes, and heart disease.

Lack of sleep, on the other hand, has numerous negative effects on the body and mind. It impairs memory, attention, and decision-making abilities, and increases the risk of depression and anxiety. Chronic sleep deprivation also contributes to weight gain and increases the risk of developing chronic health problems.

Tips for Getting Better Sleep

1. Stick to a regular sleep schedule: Try to go to bed and wake up at the same time every day, even on weekends. This helps regulate the body's circadian rhythm, which controls the sleep-wake cycle.

2. Create a sleep-conducive
   environment: Make your bedroom
   cool, dark, and quiet. Use heavy
   curtains or an eye mask to block out
   light, and invest in a comfortable
   mattress and pillows.

3. Avoid screens before bedtime: The
   blue light emitted by electronic
   devices such as phones, laptops, and
   televisions can interfere with the
   production of the sleep hormone
   melatonin, making it harder to fall
   asleep.

4. Avoid caffeine and alcohol: Caffeine is
   a stimulant that can keep you awake,
   while alcohol disrupts the quality of
   sleep. Try to avoid consuming these
   substances at least six hours before
   bedtime.

5. Exercise regularly: Regular physical
   activity can help improve the quality

of sleep, but avoid exercising too close to bedtime as it can interfere with falling asleep.

6. Establish a relaxing bedtime routine: Engage in a relaxing activity such as reading, taking a warm bath, or listening to calming music before bed. This helps signal to the brain that it is time to wind down.

In conclusion, sleep plays an important role in overall health and well-being. By following these tips, you can improve the quality and quantity of your sleep, leading to a happier, healthier life. Remember, a good night's sleep is not just a luxury but a necessity for optimal health and wellness.

Chapter 5: **Techniques for managing stress, including mindfulness and self-care practices**

Stress is a natural part of life and can arise from many sources, such as work, relationships, financial worries, and health issues. It's important to learn techniques for managing stress effectively to maintain physical, mental, and emotional well-being. This article will explore mindfulness and self-care practices that can help reduce stress levels and promote overall health and wellness.

Mindfulness:
Mindfulness is a technique that involves focusing one's attention on the present moment and accepting feelings and thoughts without judgment. Research has shown that practicing mindfulness regularly can help reduce stress levels, improve mood,

and increase resilience. Here are some simple mindfulness techniques to try:

1. Meditation: Meditation is a form of mindfulness that involves focusing the mind on a particular object, sound, or activity. It can help reduce stress levels and improve emotional regulation.

2. Deep breathing: Taking slow, deep breaths can help calm the mind and body in the face of stress. Try taking three slow breaths, holding each one for a count of five, and then exhaling slowly.

3. Body scan: The body scan involves paying attention to each part of the body, from the toes to the head, and releasing any tension or stress.

4. Gratitude journaling: Writing down things you are grateful for can help

shift your focus from negative
thoughts and feelings to positive ones,
reducing stress levels.

Self-Care Practices:
Self-care refers to activities that promote
physical, mental, and emotional well-being.
Incorporating self-care practices into your
daily routine can help reduce stress levels
and improve overall health. Here are some
self-care practices to try:

1. Exercise: Exercise is a great way to
    release stress and tension, improve
    mood, and boost energy levels. Aim to
    get at least 30 minutes of physical
    activity each day.

2. Sleep: Getting enough sleep is crucial
    for reducing stress and promoting
    overall health. Aim for 7-9 hours of
    sleep each night.

3. Healthy eating: Eating a well-balanced diet that includes plenty of fruits, vegetables, whole grains, and lean proteins can help improve mood, reduce stress levels, and boost energy levels.

4. Relaxation techniques: Relaxation techniques such as yoga, tai chi, or massage can help reduce stress levels and improve physical and emotional well-being.

In conclusion, mindfulness and self-care practices are effective techniques for managing stress. Incorporating these practices into your daily routine can help reduce stress levels, improve mood, and promote overall health and wellness. By adopting healthy habits, you can improve your quality of life and achieve optimal health and wellness.

Chapter 6: **The impact of positive thinking and mindset on physical and mental well-being**

Positive thinking and a healthy mindset can have a profound impact on our physical and mental well-being. Our thoughts, beliefs, and attitudes have the power to shape our reality and influence our health in meaningful ways. In this chapter of "Healthy Habits for a Better Life: A comprehensive guide to achieving optimal health and wellness," we will explore the ways in which positive thinking can enhance our health and well-being.

The power of positive thinking is rooted in its ability to release stress and reduce anxiety. Negative thoughts and stress have been linked to various health problems such as high blood pressure, heart disease, and weakened immune systems. On the other hand, positive thinking has been shown to reduce stress, boost the immune system, and promote overall physical and mental health.

Positive thinking can also improve our mental well-being by increasing self-esteem and reducing feelings of depression and anxiety. When we focus on positive thoughts and experiences, we are more likely to feel good about ourselves and our lives, which can lead to greater feelings of happiness and contentment.

Moreover, a positive mindset can also play a crucial role in helping us achieve our goals and overcome obstacles. By focusing on positive outcomes and visualization techniques, we can tap into the power of our subconscious minds to help us manifest our desires and reach our goals more easily.

In conclusion, positive thinking and a healthy mindset can have a profound impact on our physical and mental well-being. By focusing on positive thoughts and experiences, reducing stress, and tapping into the power of our subconscious minds, we can enhance our health and well-being and achieve our goals with ease. By incorporating positive thinking and a healthy mindset into our daily lives, we can create a life filled with happiness, success, and optimal health.

Chapter 7: **How to create a self-care routine and prioritize self-care activities**

Self-care is a crucial aspect of leading a healthy and fulfilling life. It involves taking the time to care for your physical, emotional, mental, and spiritual well-being. In this article, we'll outline the steps you need to take to create a self-care routine and prioritize self-care activities in your daily life.

1. Identify your needs: The first step in creating a self-care routine is to identify what you need to care for yourself. This can include physical, emotional, mental, and spiritual aspects of your well-being. Make a list of self-care activities that you find most beneficial and prioritize these activities.

2. Make time for self-care: The next step
    is to make time for self-care activities.
    This can be challenging, especially if
    you have a busy schedule. However,
    it's essential to set aside time each day
    for self-care. Consider waking up
    early, setting aside time in the
    evenings, or taking a break during
    your lunch hour.

3. Incorporate self-care into your daily
    routine: Once you have identified your
    needs and set aside time for self-care,
    it's essential to incorporate self-care
    activities into your daily routine. This
    could mean making a to-do list,
    scheduling self-care activities in your
    calendar, or simply finding ways to
    integrate self-care into your daily
    tasks.

4. Be consistent: Consistency is key to
    making self-care a habit. Make a
    commitment to yourself to prioritize

self-care each day and stick to your routine. This will help you feel better and more fulfilled in the long run.

5. Reevaluate and adjust: Finally, it's important to reevaluate and adjust your self-care routine regularly. As your needs and priorities change, your self-care routine should change as well. Don't be afraid to try new self-care activities and eliminate those that are no longer serving you.

In conclusion, creating a self-care routine and prioritizing self-care activities is an essential part of leading a healthy and fulfilling life. By following these steps, you can start taking care of yourself and improve your overall well-being. Remember to be consistent, flexible, and to always prioritize your self-care needs.

Chapter 8: **The importance of community and social support in maintaining healthy habits**

Introduction

In today's fast-paced world, it can be difficult to maintain healthy habits and stay on track with a healthy lifestyle. However, having a supportive community and a strong social network can greatly increase the chances of success. Research has shown that social support plays a crucial role in promoting healthy behaviors and habits, and can be a powerful tool for maintaining good health and wellness.

The Power of Community

Community and social support can provide motivation and accountability, helping individuals stick to their healthy habits and goals. When surrounded by people who share similar values and goals, individuals are more likely to feel encouraged and inspired to continue with their healthy habits. Additionally, being part of a community can provide a sense of belonging, reducing feelings of isolation and loneliness that can often undermine healthy behaviors.

Community support can also provide practical resources and information, such as tips and advice for healthy living. For example, individuals can join a fitness group, attend a health-focused workshop, or participate in a local health challenge to gain access to expert knowledge and resources that can help them maintain their healthy habits.

The Benefits of Social Support

Social support can also help individuals overcome challenges and setbacks. For example, having a supportive friend or family member to talk to during a difficult time can help individuals maintain their healthy habits and stay focused on their goals. Social support can also provide encouragement during times of stress or frustration, helping individuals stay motivated and on track.

Furthermore, social support can help individuals develop a positive self-image, which is essential for maintaining healthy habits. When individuals receive positive feedback and recognition for their healthy habits, they are more likely to feel confident and empowered, leading to a higher likelihood of continued success.

Conclusion

In conclusion, community and social support are vital components of maintaining healthy habits and achieving optimal health and wellness. Having a supportive community and social network can provide motivation, accountability, resources, and support to help individuals stick to their healthy habits and reach their goals. Whether it's through fitness groups, health workshops, or simply having a supportive friend, taking advantage of the power of community and social support is an essential step in maintaining a healthy and fulfilling life.

Chapter 9: **Strategies for staying motivated and maintaining healthy habits over time**

Introduction

Maintaining healthy habits over time can be a challenge, especially when faced with obstacles or setbacks. However, staying motivated and committed to a healthy lifestyle is essential for achieving and maintaining good health and wellness. In this article, we will explore strategies for staying motivated and maintaining healthy habits over time.

Set Specific, Achievable Goals

One of the most effective ways to stay motivated is by setting specific, achievable goals. Start by setting achievable and measurable goals, such as "I want to exercise for 30 minutes, three times a week." Having clear, attainable goals makes it easier to track progress and stay motivated, as individuals can see the tangible results of their efforts.

Track Progress and Celebrate Wins

Tracking progress and celebrating small wins can help individuals stay motivated and committed to their healthy habits. Keeping a record of daily or weekly activities, such as steps taken, meals consumed, or workouts completed, can help individuals see their progress over time and make any necessary adjustments to their routines. Celebrating small wins, such as hitting a new personal record or completing a challenging workout, can provide a sense of accomplishment and increase motivation to continue.

Find an Accountability Partner

Having an accountability partner, such as a friend or family member, can also be a powerful tool for staying motivated and maintaining healthy habits over time. An accountability partner can provide encouragement, support, and a sense of obligation to stay on track. Additionally, participating in healthy activities together, such as workout sessions or meal planning, can make the experience more enjoyable and provide a sense of community.

Get Creative

Staying motivated over time can be challenging, especially if individuals find themselves stuck in a routine. To stay motivated, it is important to get creative and find new ways to approach healthy habits. For example, trying a new workout class, trying a new recipe, or exploring a new trail can add excitement and variety to healthy habits and keep motivation levels high.

Conclusion

Maintaining healthy habits over time requires motivation and commitment, but it is achievable with the right strategies in place. By setting specific, achievable goals, tracking progress, celebrating wins, finding an accountability partner, and getting creative, individuals can stay motivated and maintain their healthy habits over the long term. By making healthy habits a part of their daily routines, individuals can enjoy the numerous benefits of a healthy lifestyle and achieve optimal health and wellness.

Chapter 10: **The role of technology and digital tools in tracking and promoting healthy habits**

Introduction

In today's digital age, technology and digital tools play a significant role in tracking and promoting healthy habits. From wearable fitness trackers to smartphone health apps, technology has made it easier for individuals to monitor their health and wellness and make positive changes to their habits. In this article, we will explore the role of technology and digital tools in tracking and promoting healthy habits.

Tracking Progress

One of the most significant advantages of technology and digital tools is the ability to track progress and monitor habits in real-time. Wearable fitness trackers, for example, can track physical activity levels, monitor heart rate, and calculate calories burned. Health apps, such as food and nutrition trackers, can help individuals monitor their calorie intake and make healthier food choices. By tracking progress and monitoring habits, individuals can identify areas where they need to make improvements and make changes to their routines to achieve their goals.

Setting Reminders

Another benefit of technology and digital tools is the ability to set reminders and automate healthy habits. For example, individuals can set reminders to drink water regularly, to take their vitamins, or to go for a walk during a break. These reminders can help individuals maintain healthy habits and make them a part of their daily routine. Additionally, many health apps have features that allow individuals to set goals and track their progress, helping them stay motivated and committed to their healthy habits.

Access to Information and Resources

Technology and digital tools also provide individuals with access to a wealth of information and resources that can help promote healthy habits. For example, health and wellness websites, online forums, and social media groups can provide information on healthy living, nutrition, and exercise. Additionally, digital tools can provide access to online workout classes, healthy recipes, and personalized nutrition plans, making it easier for individuals to adopt and maintain healthy habits.

Conclusion

In conclusion, technology and digital tools play a significant role in tracking and promoting healthy habits. By providing individuals with the ability to track progress, set reminders, and access information and resources, technology and digital tools have made it easier for individuals to adopt and maintain healthy habits. By utilizing these tools, individuals can achieve greater success in their efforts to maintain good health and wellness and lead a healthier, more fulfilling life..

www.ingramcontent.com/pod-product-compliance
Lightning Source LLC
Chambersburg PA
CBHW061607250726
48657CB00017B/2248